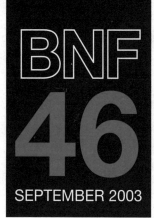

BNF
46
SEPTEMBER 2003

BNF.org

BRITISH
NATIONAL
FORMULARY

·

British Medical Association

**Royal Pharmaceutical Society
of Great Britain**

Published by the British Medical Association
Tavistock Square, London WC1H 9JP, UK
and the **Royal Pharmaceutical Society of Great Britain**
1 Lambeth High Street, London, SE1 7JN, UK
© 2003 British Medical Association and the Royal Pharmaceutical Society of Great Britain

ISBN: 0 85369 556 3 (Royal Pharmaceutical Society of Great Britain)

ISBN: 0 7279 1789 7 (British Medical Association)

ISSN: 0260-535X

Printed in Great Britain by William Clowes, Beccles, Suffolk

A catalogue record for this book is available from the British Library.

Copies may be obtained through any bookseller or direct from:

Pharmaceutical Press
 PO Box 151
 Wallingford
 Oxon OX10 8QU
 UK
 Tel: +44 (0) 1491 829 272
 Fax: +44 (0) 1491 829 292
 E-mail: rpsgb@cabi.org
 www.pharmpress.com

BMJ Bookshop
 PO Box 295
 London WC1H 9TE
 UK
 Tel: +44 (0) 20 7383 6244
 Fax: +44 (0) 20 7383 6455
 E-mail: orders@bmjbookshop.com
 www.bmjbookshop.com

The Pharmaceutical Press also supplies the BNF in digital formats suitable for standalone use or for small networks, for use over an intranet and for use on a personal digital assistant (PDA).

NHS Responseline
General practitioners and community pharmacies in **England** can telephone the NHS Responseline for enquiries concerning the direct mailing of the *British National Formulary*
Tel: 08701 555 455

For a list of name changes required by Directive 92/27/EEC, see p. x

Contents

iv

Preface

The BNF is a joint publication of the British Medical Association and the Royal Pharmaceutical Society of Great Britain. It is published under the authority of a Joint Formulary Committee which comprises representatives of the two professional bodies and of the UK Health Departments. The BNF aims to provide doctors, pharmacists and other healthcare professionals with sound up-to-date information about the use of medicines.

The BNF includes key information on the selection, prescribing, dispensing and administration of medicines. Drugs that are generally prescribed in the UK are covered and those that are considered less suitable for prescribing are clearly identified. Little or no information is included on medicines that are promoted for purchase by the public.

Basic information about drugs is drawn from the manufacturers' product literature, from medical and pharmaceutical literature, from regulatory and professional authorities, and from the data used for pricing prescriptions. Advice on the therapeutic use of medicines and on the choice of drugs is constructed from clinical literature and reflects, wherever possible, an evaluation of the evidence. The advice also takes account of authoritative national guidelines. In addition, the Joint Formulary Committee receives expert clinical advice on all therapeutic areas, particularly those that are not yet supported by good evidence; this ensures that the BNF's recommendations are relevant to practice. Many individuals and organisations contribute towards the preparation of each edition of the BNF.

The BNF is designed as a digest for rapid reference and it may not always include all the information necessary for prescribing and dispensing. Also, less detail is given on areas such as obstetrics, malignant disease, and anaesthesia since it is expected that those undertaking treatment will have specialist knowledge and access to specialist literature. The BNF is intended to be interpreted in light of professional knowledge and it should be supplemented as necessary by specialised publications and by reference to the manufacturers' product literature. Information is also available from local medicines information services (see inside front cover).

Biannual publication allows the BNF to reflect promptly changes in product availability as well as emerging safety concerns and shifts in clinical practice. The more important changes for this edition are listed on p. viii.

The BNF is now available on the internet (http://BNF.org); the site also includes additional information of relevance to healthcare professionals dealing with medicines. Other digital versions of the BNF—including intranet versions—are produced in parallel with the paper version.

The BNF welcomes comments from healthcare professionals; such comments help to ensure that the BNF remains relevant to practice. Comments and constructive criticism should be sent to:
Executive Editor, British National Formulary,
c/o Royal Pharmaceutical Society of Great Britain,
1 Lambeth High Street, London SE1 7JN.
Email: editor@bnf.org

Acknowledgements

The Joint Formulary Committee is grateful to individuals and organisations that have provided advice and information to the BNF.

The principal contributors for this edition were:

I.H. Ahmed-Jushuf, J.M. Aitken, S.P. Allison, D.G. Arkell, M. Badminton, T.P. Baglin, P.R.J. Barnes, R.H. Behrens, D. Bowsher, M.J. Brodie, R.J. Buckley, I.F. Burgess, D.J. Burn, A.J. Camm, D.A. Chamberlain, C.E. Clarke, C. Diamond, R. Dinwiddie, P.N. Durrington, A.J. Duxbury, T.S.J. Elliott, B.G. Gazzard, A.H. Ghodse, N.J.L. Gittoes, P.J. Goadsby, E.C. Gordon-Smith, I.A. Greer, J. Guillebaud, C.H. Hawkes, C.J. Hawkey, S.H.D. Jackson, J.R. Kirwan, P.G. Kopelman, M.J.S. Langman, T.H. Lee, L. Luzzatto, K.E.L. McColl, G.M. Mead, E. Miller, J.M. Neuberger, J. Nooney, D. Nutt, D.J. Oliver, L.P. Ormerod, P.A. Poole-Wilson, P.A. Routledge, D.J. Rowbotham, P.C. Rubin, R.S. Sawers, R.C. Spencer, I. Stockley, A.E. Tattersfield, H. Thomas, S. Thomas, G.R. Thompson, D.G. Waller, D.A. Warrell, A. Wilcock.

Members of the British Association of Dermatologists Therapy Guidelines and Audit Subcommittee, N.H. Cox, A.S. Highet, M.J.D. Goodfield, R.H. Meyrick-Thomas, A.D. Ormerod, J.K.L. Schofield, C.H. Smith, J.C. Sterling, and D.E. Senner (Secretariat) have provided valuable advice.

The Joint British Societies' Coronary Risk Prediction Charts have been reproduced with the kind permission of P.N. Durrington who has also provided the BNF with access to the computer program for assessing coronary and stroke risk.

Correspondents in the pharmaceutical industry have provided information on new products and commented on products in the BNF. The Prescription Pricing Authority has supplied the prices of products in the BNF.

Numerous doctors, pharmacists, nurses and others have sent comments and suggestions.

The BNF has valuable access to the *Martindale* data banks by courtesy of S. Sweetman and staff.

C.L. Iskander and R.K. Malde provided considerable assistance during the production of this edition of the BNF.

Additional checks on the BNF data were undertaken by A. Breewood, S. Coleman, M.J. Gilmour, E. Laughton, N.J. Morris and E. Rees Evans.

E.I. Connor and K.A. Parsons have assisted with the development of the electronic BNF and publishing software. Xpage and CSW Informatics Ltd have provided technical assistance with the editorial database and typesetting software.

Joint Formulary Committee 2002–2003

Chairman
Martin J. Kendall
MB, ChB, MD, FRCP

Deputy Chairman
Nicholas L. Wood
BPharm, FRPharmS

Committee Members
Peter R. Arlett
BSc, MB BS, MRCP

Alison Blenkinsopp
PhD, BPharm, FRPharmS

Peter Clappison
MB, ChB, MRCGP

Michael J. Goodman
BMBCh, BA, MA, DPhil, MRCP, FRCP

Margaret L. Hewetson
BPharm, DipHospPharm, MRPharmS

Frank P. Marsh
MA, MB, BChir, FRCP

Roopendra K. Prasad
MB BS, MS, FRCS, FRCGP

Jane Richards
OBE, MB BS, MRCS, LRCP, FRCGP, D(Obst) RCOG, DCH

James Smith
BPharm, PhD, FRPharmS, MCPP, MIInfSc

Joint Secretaries
Robert B.K. Broughton
OBE, OStJ, MB, BCh, DMRD, MHSM

Philip E. Green
BSc, MSc, LLM, MRPharmS

Executive Secretary
Lynn Clifton

Editorial Staff

Executive Editor
Dinesh K. Mehta
BPharm, MSc, FRPharmS

Senior Assistant Editor
John Martin
BPharm, PhD, MRPharmS

Assistant Editors
Bryony Jordan
BSc, DipPharmPract, MRPharmS

Colin R. Macfarlane
BPharm, MSc, MRPharmS

Rachel S. M. Ryan
BPharm, MRPharmS

Shama M. S. Wagle
BPharm, DipPharmPract, MRPharmS

Staff Editors
Fauziah T. Hashmi
BSc, MSc, MRPharmS

Sangeeta Kakar
BSc, MRPharmS

Maria Kouimtzi
BPharm, PhD, MRPharmS

Dawud Masieh
BPharm, MRPharmS

Vinaya K. Sharma
BPharm, MSc, MRPharmS

Rob Ticehurst
BSc, MRPharmS

Editorial Assistant
Gerard P. Gallagher

Head of Publishing Services
John Wilson

Director of Publications
Charles Fry

How to use the BNF

Notes on conditions, drugs and preparations

The main text consists of classified notes on clinical conditions, drugs and preparations. These notes are divided into 15 chapters, each of which is related to a particular system of the body or to an aspect of medical care. Each chapter is then divided into sections which begin with appropriate *notes for prescribers*. These notes are intended to provide information to doctors, pharmacists, nurses, and other healthcare professionals to facilitate the selection of suitable treatment. The notes are followed by details of relevant drugs and preparations.

Guidance on prescribing

This part includes information on prescription writing, controlled drugs and dependence, prescribing for children and the elderly, and prescribing in palliative care. Advice is given on the reporting of adverse reactions.

DRUG NAME ◢ ●

Indications: details of uses and indications

Cautions: details of precautions required (with cross-references to appropriate Appendixes) and also any monitoring required

COUNSELLING. Verbal explanation to the patient of specific details of the drug treatment (e.g. posture when taking a medicine)

Contra-indications: details of any contra-indications to use of drug

Side-effects: details of common and more serious side-effects

Dose: dose and frequency of administration (max. dose). CHILD and ELDERLY details of dose for specific age group

By alternative route, dose and frequency

● **Approved Name** (Non-proprietary) PoM ●
Pharmaceutical form, colour, coating, active ingredient and amount in dosage form, net price, pack size = basic NHS price. Label: (as in Appendix 9)

Proprietary Name® (Manufacturer) PoM
NHS ●
Pharmaceutical form, sugar-free, active ingredient mg/mL, net price, pack size = basic NHS price. Label: (as in Appendix 9)
Excipients: includes clinically important excipients or electrolytes
* exceptions to the prescribing status indicated by a footnote.
Note. Specific notes about the product e.g. handling

Preparations

Preparations usually follow immediately after the drug which is their main ingredient.

Preparations are included under a non-proprietary title, if they are marketed under such a title, if they are not otherwise prescribable under the NHS, or if they may be prepared extemporaneously.

If proprietary preparations are of a distinctive colour this is stated.

In the case of compound preparations the indications, cautions, contra-indications, side-effects, and interactions of all constituents should be taken into account for prescribing.

Emergency treatment of poisoning

This chapter provides information on the management of acute poisoning when first seen in the home, although aspects of hospital-based treatment are mentioned.

Appendixes and indexes

The appendixes include information on interactions, liver disease, renal impairment, pregnancy, breast-feeding, intravenous additives, borderline substances, wound management products, and cautionary and advisory labels for dispensed medicines. They are designed for use in association with the main body of the text.

The Dental Practitioners' List and the Nurse Prescribers' List are also included in this section. The indexes consist of the Index of Manufacturers and the Main Index.

Drugs

Drugs appear under pharmacopoeial or other non-proprietary titles. When there is an *appropriate current monograph* (Medicines Act 1968, Section 65) preference is given to a name at the head of that monograph; otherwise a British Approved Name (BAN), if available, is used (see also p. x).

The symbol ◢ is used to denote those preparations that are considered by the Joint Formulary Committee to be less suitable for prescribing. Although such preparations may not be considered as drugs of first choice, their use may be justifiable in certain circumstances.

Prescription-only medicines PoM

This symbol has been placed against those preparations that are available only on medical or dental prescription. For more detailed information see *Medicines, Ethics and Practice*, No. 27, London, Pharmaceutical Press, 2003 (and subsequent editions as available).

The symbol CD indicates that the preparation is subject to the prescription requirements of the Misuse of Drugs Act. For regulations governing prescriptions for such preparations see pages 7–9.

Preparations not available for NHS prescription NHS

This symbol has been placed against those preparations included in the BNF that are not prescribable under the NHS. Those prescribable only for specific disorders have a footnote specifying the condition(s) for which the preparation remains available. Some preparations which are not *prescribable* by brand name under the NHS may nevertheless be *dispensed* using the brand name providing that the prescription shows an appropriate non-proprietary name.

Prices

Prices have been calculated from the basic cost used in pricing NHS prescriptions dispensed in May 2003 or later, see p. vii for further details.

Patient Packs

On January 1 1994, Directive 92/27/EEC came into force, giving the requirements for the labelling of medicines and outlining the format and content of patient information leaflets to be supplied with every medicine. The directive also requires the use of Recommended International Non-proprietary Names for drugs (see p. x).

All medicines have approved labelling and patient information leaflets; anyone who supplies a medicine is responsible for providing the relevant information to the patient (see also Appendix 9).

Many medicines are available in manufacturers' original packs complete with patient information leaflets. Where patient packs are available, the BNF shows the number of dose units in the packs. In particular clinical circumstances, where patient packs need to be split or medicines are provided in bulk dispensing packs, manufacturers will provide additional supplies of patient information leaflets on request.

During the revision of each edition of the BNF careful note is taken of the information that appears on the patient information leaflets. Where it is considered appropriate to alert a prescriber to some specific limitation appearing on the patient information leaflet (for example, in relation to pregnancy) this advice now appears in the BNF.

The patient information leaflet also includes details of all inactive ingredients in the medicine. A list of common E numbers and the inactive ingredients to which they correspond is now therefore included in the BNF (see inside back cover).

PACT and SPA

PACT (Prescribing Analyses and Cost) and SPA (Scottish Prescribing Analysis) provide prescribers with information about their prescribing.

The *PACT Standard Report*, or in Scotland SPA *Level 1 Report*, is sent to all general practitioners on a quarterly basis. It contains an analysis of the practitioner's prescribing over the last 3 months, and for a given topic of prescribing, it compares the individual practice with the Health Authority equivalents.

The *PACT Catalogue*, or in Scotland SPA *Level 2 Report*, provides a full inventory of the prescriptions issued by a prescriber. The PACT catalogue is available on request for periods between 1 and 24 months. To allow the prescriber to target specific areas of prescribing, a Catalogue may be requested to cover individual preparations, BNF sections, or combinations of BNF chapters.

PACT is also available electronically. This system gives users on-line access through NHSnet to the 3 years' prescribing data held on the Prescription Pricing Authority's database.

Prices in the BNF

Basic **net prices** are given in the BNF to provide an indication of relative cost. Where there is a choice of suitable preparations for a particular disease or condition the relative cost may be used in making a selection. Cost-effective prescribing must, however, take into account other factors (such as dose frequency and duration of treatment) that affect the total cost. The use of more expensive drugs is justified if it will result in better treatment of the patient or a reduction of the length of an illness or the time spent in hospital.

Prices have generally been calculated from the net cost used in pricing NHS prescriptions dispensed in May 2003, but where available later prices have been included; unless an original pack is available these prices are based on the largest pack size of the preparation in use in community pharmacies. The price for an extemporaneously prepared preparation has been omitted where the net cost of the ingredients used to make it would give a misleadingly low impression of the final price. In Appendix 8 prices stated are per dressing or bandage.

The unit of 20 is still sometimes used as a basis for comparison, but where suitable original packs or patient packs are available these are priced instead.

Gross prices vary as follows:

1. Costs to the NHS are greater than the net prices quoted and include professional fees and overhead allowances;
2. Private prescription charges are calculated on a separate basis;
3. Over-the-counter sales are at retail price, as opposed to basic net price, and include VAT.

BNF prices are NOT, therefore, suitable for quoting to patients seeking private prescriptions or contemplating over-the-counter purchases.

A fuller explanation of costs to the NHS may be obtained from the Drug Tariff.

It should be noted that separate Drug Tariffs are applicable to England and Wales, Scotland, and Northern Ireland. Prices in the different tariffs may vary.

Changes for this edition

Significant changes

The BNF is revised twice yearly and numerous changes are made between issues. All copies of BNF No. 45 (March 2003) should therefore be withdrawn and replaced by BNF No. 46 (September 2003). Significant changes have been made in the following sections for BNF No. 46:

Combined use of aspirin and clopidogrel [updated advice], section 2.9

Hypothyroidism and lipid-regulating drugs [new text], section 2.12

Statins [revised text], section 2.12

Drugs for asthma in breast-feeding [updated advice], section 3.1

Cromoglicate and related therapy [updated advice], section 3.3.1

Drugs used in Parkinsonism [revised text], section 4.9

Dopaminergic drugs used in Parkinsonism [revised text], section 4.9.1

Antimuscarinic drugs used in Parkinsonism [revised text], section 4.9.2

Paroxetine not recommended for depression in those under 18 years [CSM advice], section 4.3.3

Antibacterial treatment of incubating syphilis [new text], Table 1, section 5.1

Antibacterial treatment of uncomplicated gonorrhoea [revised text], Table 1, section 5.1

Antibacterial treatment of osteomyelitis and septic arthritis [revised text], Table 1, section 5.1

Antibacterial treatment of septicaemia related to vascular catheter [revised text], Table 1, section 5.1

Antibacterial treatment of otitis media [revised text], Table 1, section 5.1

Antibacterial treatment of throat infections [revised text], Table 1, section 5.1

Management of anthrax [revised text], section 5.1.12

Capecitabine and tegafur with uracil for metastatic colorectal cancer [NICE guidance], section 8.1.3

Capecitabine for locally advanced or metastatic breast cancer [NICE guidance], section 8.1.3

Use of irradiated blood products with cladrabine and fludarabine [new text], section 8.1.3

Control of microbial contamination of eye preparations [updated advice], section 11.2

Topical pimecrolimus and tacrolimus for atopic eczema [updated advice], section 13.5.3

Meningococcal vaccine for travellers [updated advice], section 14.4

Nephrotoxicity associated with interaction between sevoflurane and carbon dioxide absorbents [new text], section 15.1.2

Dose changes

Changes in dose statements introduced into BNF No. 46:

Amoxicillin [anthrax], p. 261
Caspofungin, p. 295
Ceftazidime, p. 268
Celecoxib, p. 482
Chlorambucil, p. 411
Clozapine, p. 180
Erythromycin [pertussis prevention], p. 275
Etodolac, p. 484
Etomidate-Lipuro®, p. 603
Hypnomidate®, p. 603
Melphalan, p. 412
Prednisolone [daily dose for myasthenia gravis], p. 500
Procaine Benzylpenicillin [for syphilis], p. 255
Tranexamic Acid, p. 122
Viazem XL®, p. 103

Classification changes

Classification changes have been made in the following sections for BNF No. 46:

Section 2.12 Ezetimibe [new subsection]

Section 6.4.1.1 Women with uterus [subsection no longer exists]

Section 6.4.1.1 Women without a uterus [subsection no longer exists]

Section 6.7.1 Bromocriptine and other dopaminergic drugs [title change]

Section 7.3.1 Combined hormonal contraceptives [title change]

Section 7.4.5 Phosphodiesterase type-5 inhibitors [subtitle change]

Section 14.4 Measles, Mumps and Rubella (MMR) vaccine [subtitle change]

New names

Name changes introduced into BNF No. 46 (see also p. x):

Asacol® *MR* [formerly *Asacol*®], p. 48
Actrapid [formerly *Human Actrapid*®], p. 330
Insulatard® [formerly *Human Insulatard*®], p. 331
Lyrinel® *XL* [formerly *Ditropan*® *XL*], p. 401
Mixtard® *10* [formerly *Human Mixtard*® *10*], p. 332
Mixtard® *20* [formerly *Human Mixtard*® *20*], p. 332
Mixtard® *30* [formerly *Human Mixtard*® *30*], p. 332
Mixtard® *40* [formerly *Human Mixtard*® *40*], p. 333
Mixtard® *50* [formerly *Human Mixtard*® *50*], p. 333
Monotard® [formerly *Human Monotard*®], p. 331
Ultratard® [formerly *Human Ultratard*®], p. 331
Velosulin® [formerly *Human Velosulin*®], p. 330